Ahmed HARBAOUI

Management of intracranial subdural empyema

Ahmed HARBAOUI

Management of intracranial subdural empyema

Epidemiology and treatment

ScienciaScripts

Cover image: www.ingimage.com

This book is a translation from the original published under ISBN 978-620-6-72215-1.

Publisher:
Sciencia Scripts
is a trademark of
Dodo Books Indian Ocean Ltd. and OmniScriptum S.R.L publishing group

120 High Road, East Finchley, London, N2 9ED, United Kingdom
Str. Armeneasca 28/1, office 1, Chisinau MD-2012, Republic of Moldova, Europe
Printed at: see last page
ISBN: 978-620-8-25078-2

TABLE OF CONTENTS

INTRODUCTION 2

PATIENTS AND METHODS 3

RESULTS 7

DISCUSSION...24

CONCLUSIONS 49

BIBLIOGRAPHICAL REFERENCES 54

INTRODUCTION

Intracranial suppurations are relatively rare but can be potentially serious and life-threatening. Intracranial empyema (ICPE), which is a collection of pus within the natural intracranial spaces, accounts for 31 to 65% of cases, depending on the series published [1]. Subdural empyema, which develops in the subdural space (between the dura mater and the arachnoid), is the most common location for intracranial empyema (CTE), and is most often associated with a pyogenic infection. It is a genuine medical and surgical emergency [2].

The advent of new imaging techniques has made it possible to diagnose intracranial subdural empyema (ISCDE) earlier, with greater topographical accuracy and better management, thereby improving prognosis and reducing neurological sequelae.

A number of authors have adopted a primarily medical approach to the treatment of CTE, and in particular ESDTC, based essentially on antibiotic therapy, reserving surgery for a few special cases. However, few studies have been carried out on ESDTCs over the last ten years, and there is no consensus on their therapeutic management once the diagnosis has been made [1, 2, 3].

In our work, we reported the experience of the neurosurgery department of the Tunis Military Hospital by analysing the different parameters collected on 53 cases of ESDTC admitted over a period of 15 years (January 2000 to December 2014).

We studied and analysed the epidemiological, clinical and neuroradiological data, the diagnostic problems, the contribution of complementary examinations, the therapeutic attitudes and the evolutionary consequences, comparing our results with those of the literature, in order to propose a standardised management of ESDTC with pyogenic germs in immunocompetent adults.

PATIENTS AND METHODS

1. Type of study :

We conducted a retrospective study including 53 patients who presented with ESDTC and were hospitalised in the neurosurgery department of the Tunis Military Hospital over a 15-year period from January 2000 to December 2014. The different cases were identified from the handwritten and electronic archives of the department, as well as the handwritten archives of the operating theatre.

2. Inclusion criteria :

- Neuroimaging suggestive of ESDTC.
- Age 2: 15 years.
- Pyogenic germ isolated / no germ isolated on bacteriological sample(s).
- No history of immunodepression or cranioencephalic surgery, in particular evacuation of a chronic subdural haematoma.

3. Exclusion criteria :

- Appearance suggestive of other intracranial suppuration on neuroimaging (cerebral abscess, extra-dural empyema).
- Cerebral empyema caused by fungi, parasites and tuberculosis.
- Age < 15 years.
- Context of immunodepression.
- Patients who benefited surgery including evacuation of a chronic subdural haematoma.

4. Survey procedures :

The data collected was transcribed onto Microsoft Office Excel 200?

4.1. Epidemiological data :

Annual frequency, age, sex.

4.2. Etiological data :

- Local or contiguous infection.
- Infection by direct plating.
- Entrance unknown.

4.3. Clinical data :

Mode of onset, duration of symptoms, clinical signs. (HTTC, infectious syndrome, vigilance disorder, meningeal signs, focal neurological signs), clinical forms (typical forms and pauci-symptomatic forms).

4.4. Para-clinical data :

- Radiological data: cerebral CT and MRI scans
- Biological data: CBC, ESR, CRP
- Bacteriological data: Pus from the empyema, sampling at the site of entry, lumbar puncture (LP).

4.5. Therapeutic data :

4.5.1. Curative treatment :

- Treatment medical exclusive / Treatment surgical treatment.
- Medical treatment: a combination of broad-spectrum antibiotics.
- Treatment surgical (trepanation/craniectomy or craniotomy).

4.5.2. Symptomatic treatment :

- Anti-oedematous treatment.
- Anti-epileptic treatment.

4.5.3. Treatment of the front door

4.6. Data from inpatient monitoring :

Clinical, biological and radiological parameters.

4.7. Evolving data :

The evolution a has been categorized as favourable and unfavourable.

- Patients were considered to have had a favourable outcome if they showed clinical improvement (regression of signs of intracranial hypertension, improvement in the state of consciousness, return to apyrexia in the event of fever) and radiological improvement (reduction in the size of the empyema, reduction in peri-lesional oedema, reduction in the mass effect), with normal autonomy at discharge, whether or not associated with the existence of a moderate disability (GOS=4 - 5).
- Patients who died during hospitalisation, or who presented a severe disability at discharge with loss of autonomy, despite clinical and radiological improvement, were considered to have had an unfavourable outcome (GOS=1 to 3).

4.8. Follow-up data after discharge :

The various clinical parameters (presence or absence of disability, presence or absence of improvement or worsening of disability, presence or absence of signs of recurrence of empyema), scans, etc. (time to 1[er] check-up after discharge, CT appearance, number of examinations) and therapeutic (treatment in progress, duration, whether or not treatment of the portal of entry was carried out) follow-up at the neurosurgery outpatient clinic were collected and studied, with a 2-year follow-up.

5. Statistical analysis :

We performed a univariate statistical analysis using Fisher's exact test and the Odd-ratio, comparing the 2 groups of patients (favourable evolution / unfavourable evolution) according to the following factors:

- Age
- Gender
- Duration of symptoms
- Initial state of consciousness (arbitrarily divided into 2 groups: GCS< 12/15 and GCS> 12/15)
- Siege of the empyema

- Entrance door
- Surgical technique

Significance was retained for a value of $p<0.05$.

RESULTS

1. Epidemiological data :

1.1. Frequency :

Over a period of 15 years, the department recorded 53 cases of ESDTC, representing a frequency of 3.53 cases/year.

Table T: Breakdown of patients by year

Year	Number of cases
2000	6
2001	4
2002	2
2003	1
2004	6
2005	2
2006	5
2007	5
2008	2
2009	6
2010	4
2011	2
2012	5
2013	1
2014	2

1.2. Breakdown by age :

The average age was 41.5, with extremes of 15 and 68. The breakdown by 10-year age group showed a predominance of the 15-25 age group (29 cases, or 54.5%).

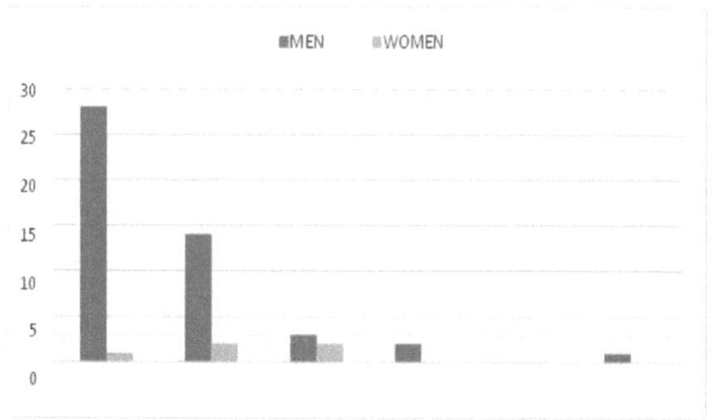

Figure 1: Breakdown of cases by age group and sex

1.3. Breakdown by gender :

There was a clear male predominance, with a sex ratio of 9.6.

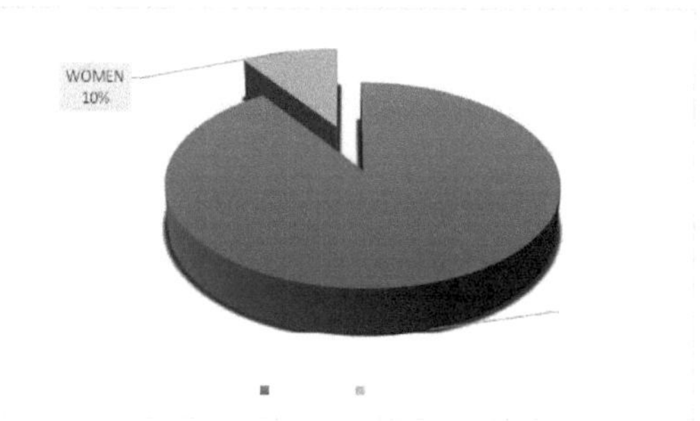

Figure 2: Breakdown of patients by gender

2. Aetiological data :

Table TT: Breakdown of patients by aetiology

Causes	Percentage
Locoregional infection	83% (44/53)
Infection by sowing	1,9% (1/53)
Entry door unknown	15,1% (8/53)

2.1. Local or contiguous infection :

Locoregional infection is the most common aetiology: 83%.

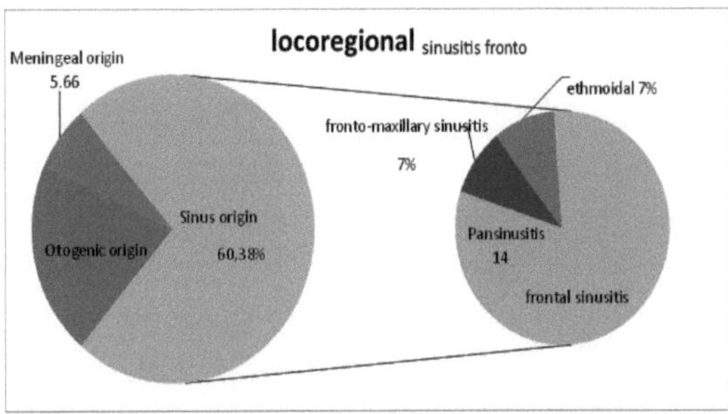

Figure 3: Origin of locoregional infections

2.2. Infection by direct plating :

1 case of neglected craniocerebral wound was found, representing 1.9% of cases.

2.3. Entry door unknown :

In 8 patients, no portal of entry was found, i.e. 15.1% of cases. The majority (8?.5%) underwent a full systematic aetiological work-up including cardiac ultrasound, blood cultures and an ENT and stomatology consultation. In 6 cases (?5%), HTV serology was carried out and found to be negative.

3. Clinical data :

3.1. Mode of installation :

In the majority of patients (90.5%), the clinical picture had developed progressively or rapidly. Brutality of symptoms was observed in 5 cases (9.4%) of patients with inaugural comititude.

3.2. Duration of symptoms :

Varying from a few days to a few weeks, the average was 9 days, with a maximum of 2 months and a minimum of 3 days.

Table TTT: Duration of symptoms in our series

Duration of	ESDIC(n=53)	
symptoms (weeks)	Number	Percentage
1	8	15,09%
1-2	41	?,36%
2-3	2	3,??%
>3	2	3,??%

In our series, symptoms predominated between 1 and 2 weeks in duration, with 92.45% of patients presenting with symptoms that had been evolving for less than 15 days.

3.3.Clinical symptoms :

3.3.1 Clinical signs :

a. Intracranial hypertension syndrome (ICHT) :

46 patients (86.8%) had presented with one or more signs of CTE. Fundus examination in 8 patients (15%) showed papilledema in 3 patients.

b. Infectious syndrome :

A fever of 38°C or higher, often associated with asthenia and anorexia, was found in 39 patients, i.e. ?3.58% of cases.

c. Impaired alertness :

Impaired vigilance was found in 48 patients (90.5% of cases).

GCS14-12 = 34 cases

GCS12-8 = 5 cases

GCS<8 = 3 cases

d. Meningeal signs :

Stiffness of the neck, whether or not associated with a Kernig and/or Brudzinski sign, was reported in 3 cases (5.66%) in the context of purulent meningitis.

e. Focal neurological signs :

Found in 24 patients (45.28%) (Table 4).
e1. Sensory-motor deficits :

- Motor impairment: 14 cases (26.41%)

► Hemiplegia: 1 case
► Hemiparesis: 12 cases
► Monoparesis: 1 case
► Hemicorporeal hyperaesthesia: 1 case (1.9%)

e2. Damage to the cranial pairs :

Found in 11 patients (20,?5%).

- Involvement of the TT: 3 cases
- Involvement of the VT: 4 cases
- Impairment of DTC: 3 cases
- ATV involvement: 1 case

e3. Language disorders :

Were present in 4 patients (?.5%).

- Phasic disorders: 3 cases
- Dysarthria: 1 case

e4. Comitial seizures :

Found in 12 cases, or 22.6%, represented by :

- Generalised convulsive seizures: ? cases
- Hemicorporeal seizures: 3 cases
- Convulsive seizures localised to an upper limb: 1 case
- Convulsive seizures localised to a lower limb: 1case

e5. Cerebellar syndrome :

Was present in 1 patient, i.e. 1.9% of cases.

e6. Frontal syndrome :

Observed in ? patients (13.2%). Tl was manifested by memory and behavioural problems.

Table TV: Breakdown of focal signs

Focusing signs	Number	Percentage
Motor deficit	14	26,41%
Comitial seizure	12	22,6%
Reaching pairs cranial	11	20,?5%
Language disorders	4	?,5%
Frontal syndrome	?	13,2%
Cerebellar syndrome	1	1,9%
Sensory disorders	1	1,9%

3.3.2. Clinical forms :

(Table V)

a- Typical form :

The classic Bergman triad (HTTC syndrome/infectious syndrome/focal neurological signs) was present in 21 patients in our series, i.e. 39.6%.

b- Pauci-symptomatic forms :

These were the most frequent forms in our series, accounting for 60.4% of cases. They were manifested by only one or two elements of Bergman's triad.

Table V: Symptomatic associations at the time of diagnosis of ESDTC

Associations symptomatic	Number of cases (n=53)	Percentage
HTTC+ST+SF	21	39,6%
HTTC+SF	11	20,?%
HTTC+ST	9	16,9%
HTTC	8	15,1%
SF	2	3,8%
ST+SF	2	3,8%

HTTC : Intracranial hypertension syndrome ST: Infectious syndrome SF: Focal signs.

4. Para-clinical data :

4.1. Radiological data :

4.1.1. Cerebral CT :

All patients underwent a first-line CT scan without and with contrast injection. Cerebral CT enabled positive diagnosis of cerebral empyema in 98.11% of cases and assessment of the location, size and various associated lesions.

a - Positive diagnosis :

In 52 cases, cerebral CT showed an image suggestive of subdural empyema: a hypodense subdural collection whose periphery was enhanced after injection of PDC, sometimes associated with an area of hypodense vasogenic cerebral oedema (8 cases, i.e. 15.1%). In only one patient, who had renal insufficiency that prevented the injection of contrast medium, was the existence of a hypodense, non-oedematogenic subdural collection insufficient to rule out a chronic subdural haematoma.

b - Headquarters :

The preferred site was supratentorial (98%,1). The posterior cerebral fossa was involved in only 1 case (1.9%). The most frequent location was frontal: 19 cases (35.85%) and hemispheric collections represented 20.5% (11 cases) (Table VT).

Table VT: Breakdown of patients by ESDTC topography

Headquarters	Number of cases	Percentage
*Sus tentoriel	52	98,1%
Front	19	35,85%
Temporal	5	9,4%
Parietal	5	9,4%
Fronto-parietal	6	11,32%
Temporo-parietal	2	3,??%
Hemispheric	11	20,?%
Tnter-hemispherique	4	?,55%
*Under tentorium	1	1,9%

c- Size :

The subdural empyema varied in size, ranging from approximately 1mm to 08mm in thickness.

d- Number :

Among the 53 cases collected in our series :

- 50 patients had a single subdural empyema.
- 2 patients had 2 subdural empyema.
- 1 patient had 3 subdural empyema.

e- Associated lesions :

(Mountain bike table)

Table VTT: Breakdown of patients by associated lesions

Associated lesions	Number of patients	Percentage affected
Commitment sub falcoriel	36	6?,9%
Sinus thrombosis sagittal	1	1,9%
Sinus thrombosis sigmoid	1	1,9%
Sinus filling	32	60,38%
Ear filling mastoid	9	16,98%
Brain abscess	1	1,9%
Traumatic lesion opposite the empyema (pneumocephalus+) subcutaneous collection)	1	1,9%

4.1.2. Cerebral MRI with diffusion sequence :

Cerebral MRI was performed in one patient (1.9% of cases). It was used to diagnose subdural empyema, showing a subdural collection with T1 hyposignal, T2 hypersignal and peripheral enhancement on injection of gadolinium, and showing diffusion restriction with a low diffusion coefficient (ADC).

4.2. Biological data :

4.2.1. Blood count (CBC) :

Carried out in all patients. The CBC showed hyperleukocytosis in 31 patients (58.5%).

4.2.2. Sedimentation rate (VS):

The SV was accelerated (greater than 10mm at 1ère hours) in 22 patients, i.e. 41.5%.

4.2.3. C reactive protein (CRP) :

Measured in 3? patients, it was elevated (above 8 mg/L) in 19 of them, or 51.35%.

4.3. Bacteriological data :

4.3.1. Pus of empyema :

The bacteriological study of the empyema pus was carried out in the 48 cases operated on in our department. The pathogen was found in 3 cases, i.e. 6.25% of the samples taken.

The germs found in our series were :

- Streptococcus milleri (Aerobic, gram-positive cocci, sinus origin): 1 case.
- Streptococcus sp (Aerobic, gram+ cocci,origin unknown):   case.
- Brevibacterium spp (Aerobic, gram+ bacillus, otogenic origin): 1 case.

The sample was sterile in 45 cases, i.e. 93.5% of samples taken.

4.3.2. Sampling at the entrance door :

Bacteriological examination of the auricular pus carried out in 8 patients came back sterile each time.

4.3.3. Lumbar puncture :

Performed on 3 patients (before they were referred to us). The results showed purulent CSF with no germs on direct examination or culture in the 3 cases.

5. Treatments :

5.1. Medical treatment :

5.1.1. Antibiotic therapy :

All patients in our series received antibiotic treatment (Table VTTT):The Cefotaxime/fosfomycin/metronidazole combination was the most widely used (69.8%).

The average duration of parenteral treatment was 34.5 days, with a minimum of 22 days and a maximum of 4? days.

It should be noted that 6 patients in our series benefited from oral relay: Ciprofloxacin in 4 cases and Rifampicin + Ciprofloxacin in 2 cases.

Table VTTT: Breakdown of patients by combination of antibiotics administered

Combination of ATBs Number of Percentage of patients (n=53)		
Cefotaxime+fosfomycin+Metronidazole	3?	69,8%
Ciprofloxacin+fosfomycin+fosfomycin Metronidazole	5	9,4%
Cefotaxime + Chloramphenicol Metronidazole	5	9,4%
Cefotaxime + Ciprofloxacin + Metronidazole	2	3,??%
Tmipenem+ Vancomycin+ Ciprofloxacin	1	1,9%
Rifampicin+ Ciprofloxacin	1	1,9%
Ciprofloxacin + Chloramphenicol + Metronidazole	1	1,9%
Fosfomycin+ Amikacin	1	1,9%

5.1.2. Others :

a - Treatment of cerebral oedema :

Our series included ? patients with cerebral oedema, i.e. 13.21% of cases. These patients received the following treatment: Dexamethasone at a dose of 8 to 12 mg/d, for a variable duration ranging from 3 to 8 days (average 5.5 days), followed by gradual tapering off over a week.

b - Anti-comital treatment :

12 patients (22.6%) had suffered a convulsive seizure, including :

- 4 patients have were put on Phenobarbital (Gardénal®).
- 3 patients were put on sodium Valproate (Depakine®).
- 5 patients have were put on Carbamazepine (Tegretol®).

5.2. Surgical treatment

5.2.1. Sickle cell /Craniectomy :

In our series, 45 patients, i.e. 84.94%, underwent surgical treatment based on trepanation +/- craniectomy. Of these, 36 patients underwent 2-hole trepanation and 3 patients underwent single-hole trepanation. Repeat surgery to re-evacuate the empyema through the trepan hole(s) was necessary in 2 of the 39 patients mentioned above. 6 patients underwent craniectomy to enlarge the trepan hole (Table TX).

Table TX: Patients who underwent trepanation +/- craniectomy

Type of surgery	Number of cases	Percentage
2-hole bit	36	6?,92%
Single-hole drill bit	3	5,66%
Craniectomy	6	11,32%

5.2.2. Craniotomy :

3 patients in our series (5.66%) underwent craniotomy to evacuate the empyema. In 2 patients, craniotomy was necessary because of a lack of clinical and radiological improvement after repeat surgery to re-evacuate the empyema through the trepan hole(s). In one patient, craniotomy was the first choice because of very dense pus that could not be evacuated through the trepan hole(s).

5.3. Therapeutic methods :

(Figure 4).

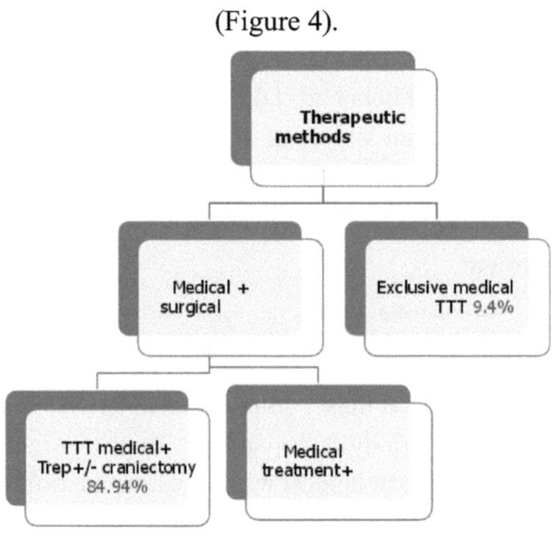

TTT: treatment; Trep: trepanation

Figure 4: Treatment modalities

In our series, the majority of patients (90.6%) received medical and surgical treatment. Only 5 patients had received exclusive medical treatment, representing 9.4% of cases (Table X).

Table X: Breakdown of patients treated by exclusive medical therapy.

Location from empyema	Number of cases	Percentage
Hemispheric inter- empyema no compressive	3	5,66%
Empyema subdural non-compressive forehead	1	1,9%
Subdural empyema of the posterior fossa fossa not compressive	1	1,9%

5.4. Treatment of the front door :

In our series, 36 of the 53 patients, i.e. 6?.92%, each benefited from therapeutic management adapted to the portal of entry of their ESDTC (Table XT).

Table XT: Distribution of patients according to therapeutic management of empyema entry sites

Front doorNumber of cases	
Sinus origin	28
Otogenic origin	4
Meningeal origin	3
Wound craniocerebral neglected	1

5.5. Monitoring during treatment :

All patients underwent daily clinical monitoring (state of consciousness, signs of HTTC, focal neurological signs, temperature) and biological monitoring (at least a bi-weekly CBC was performed in 96.24% of patients, with or without an associated VS and/or CRP). The stability or improvement of the state of consciousness, the regression of the signs of of HTTC, thermal defervescence and decreases in white blood cell count, SV and/or CRP were considered to indicate the efficacy of the treatment undertaken.

- 91.66% of patients underwent a follow-up cerebral CT scan without and with PDC injection within 24 to 48 hours of empyema evacuation.
- Non-operated subjects and stable post-operative subjects underwent a follow-up cerebral CT scan every ? to 10 days in ?1,?% of cases.

- In 96.2% of cases, the follow-up cerebral CT scan performed during the last week of hospitalisation showed: a significant reduction in the thickness of the subdural collection (:S 2mm), a clear regression or even disappearance of the cerebral oedema opposite, a reduction in peripheral contrast, and even the absence of a subdural collection.

6. Complications :

(Table XTT).

Table XTT: Distribution of patients according to complications

Complications	Manifestations	Number of case	Percentage
Brain engagement temporal	Coma Anisocoria homolateral	2	3?,?%
Sub-falcoral commitment	Disturbed alertness/focal neurological signs (inconsistent)	36	6?,9%
Thrombosis of the sagittal sinus superior		1	1,9%
Thrombosis of the left sigmoid sinus		1	1,9%
Comitiality		12	22,6%

7. Course and prognosis :

7.1. Favourable evolution:

In our series, 50 patients (94.34%) had a favourable outcome. On discharge from the neurosurgery department, they were all autonomous and capable of normal daily activity (G.O.S=5-4), including :

- 46 patients (86, ?9%) had a strictly normal neurological examination
- 4 patients (?,55%) had a minor disability (G.O.S=4) such as :

✓ Discrete haemiparesis: 2 cases

✓ Discrete monoparesis: 1 case

✓ Partial monocular palsy of the VT: 1 case

7.2. Unfavourable trend :

In our series, 3 patients, i.e. 5.66% of cases, had an unfavourable evolution: these patients died (G.O.S=1). (Table XTTT).

Table XTTT: Description of patients with an unfavourable outcome (death)

Age	Door Probable entry	Signs Clinic on admission	CT SCAN brain	Act surgery performed	Evolution
24 years old	Sinus	GCS=6/15 Left anisocoria	-Compressive left hemispheric subdural empyema -Pansinusitis	Trepanning	-Septic shock -left posterior cerebral collapse -Death at D2 hospitalisation
19 years old	Otological (history of chronic otitis media) +	GCS=4/15 Right anisocoria	-Right temporal parietal subdural empyema -Very severe cerebral oedema -Ear filling mastoid	Trepanning	-Brain death - neurovegetative disorders -death on D3 of hospitalisation
53 years old	Known	GCS=11/15	Right frontal subdural empyema	Trepanning	-Pulmonary embolism - death at D9 hospitalisation

7.3. Statistical analysis of likely prognostic factors :

(Table XTV)

7.3.1. Age :

There was no statistically significant difference in progression according to age (p=1).

7.3.2. Gender :

There was no statistically significant difference between the sexes (p=1).

7.3.3. Duration of symptoms :

There was no statistically significant difference in progression according to the duration of symptoms (p=1).

7.3.4. State of consciousness on admission (GCS) :

There was a statistically significant relationship between initial state of consciousness and outcome (P<0.01), which means that a GCS>12 on admission was significantly associated with a favourable outcome, and a GCS<12 on admission was significantly associated with an unfavourable outcome.

7.3.5. Seat of the empyema :

There was no statistically significant difference in the course of the disease depending on whether it was located above or below the tentorium (p=1).

7.3.6. Front door :

There was no statistically significant difference in outcome depending on whether or not there was a known route of entry (p=0.349).

7.3.7. Therapeutic methods :

There was no statistically significant difference in outcome according to the surgical technique used (p=1).

Table XTV: Univariate statistical analysis (Fisher exact test / Odd- Ratio)

Evolution favourable		Evolution unfavourable	P
Age> 25 years	23	1	1
Men	45	3	1
Symptoms< 15 days	46	3	1
GCS> 12	40	0	<0,01
Trepanning/ Craniectomy	42	3	1
Craniotomy	3	0	1
Sus- tentorial	49	3	1
Entrance door unknown	?	1	0,394

7.4. Follow-up and prognosis :

We collected data on patient follow-up, which was carried out at the neurosurgery consultation with a 2-year follow-up.

Of the 50 living patients discharged, 4 were lost to follow-up. The other patients all received a follow-up brain CT scan without and with injection of PDC within a month of discharge. 91.30% of patients had 2 consultations and 2 follow-up brain CT scans without and with contrast injection in the 3 months following discharge.

- 3 patients, or 6%, were referred back to ENT for further treatment of the entry site.
- 22 patients, i.e. 44%, showed complete normalisation at the 1er scan check.
- 4 patients (8%) showed an improvement in their motor deficit.
- 2 patients, or 4% (with no history of convulsions) developed comititude requiring anti-epileptic medication.
- For patients who developed comititude during hospitalisation, anti-epileptic treatment was continued for at least 1 year in ?5% of them.
- There was no recurrence of subdural empyema in any patient.

DISCUSSION

CTEs are rarer than brain abscesses, accounting for 25-31% of intracranial suppurations [1]. ESDTCs are the most common type of ETC (?5% of cases). They represent a genuine medical and surgical emergency [1, 2, 3].

I- History

The first descriptions of ESD were reported in the 18th century, with De Lapeyronie in 1?09 and Schmuker in 1??6 mentioning cases that can now be recognised as post-traumatic subdural empyema, and Richter in 1??3 describing a probable ESD secondary to frontal sinusitis [4,5].The term ESD was used by Kubik et al [6] in 1943, in preference to the less precise terms subdural suppuration, subdural abscess, intra-dural abscess, intra-arachnoid abscess, intra-meningeal abscess, internal or purulent pachymeningitis, circumscribed meningitis or phlegmonous meningitis, which have been used in turn.

There have been three periods in the management of cranioencephalic suppurations:

► The period before antibiotics (ATB) (1945): treatment of these suppurative collections was mainly surgical, involving puncture with drainage or excision. The prognosis was poor, with a high mortality rate (over 80%) [?]

► The ATB period and before the CT scan (19?5): treatment was medical (antibiotic therapy) and surgical without good topographical accuracy, with an improvement in the vital prognosis (the mortality rate fell from 80% to 30%) [...].

► The modern period, with CT scans, bacteriology and the new ATBs: topographical diagnosis has become precise, with the possibility of isolating most germs, but culture is sometimes negative even in the absence of prior antibiotic therapy. Treatment is now based on broad-spectrum antibiotic therapy and/or surgery, with an extremely significant improvement in prognosis [?]

II-Pathogenesis

ETCs are pericerebral collections that arise in the vast majority of cases from infection of the facial bone or rock. More rarely, they may also develop as a result of direct contamination through a wound or after evacuation of a subdural haematoma, for example. This collection may be extra-dural, in a space created by a pathological process detaching the dura mater from the deep planes of the bony vault [8], or sub-dural, crossing the dura mater perhaps through micro-thrombophlebitis phenomena. Thrombophlebitis, which is a serious complication of this type of cerebral infection, can be explained by the abundance of veins in this subdural space.

Bacteriologically, empyemas are caused by the same bacteria as abscesses, with a polymicrobial flora composed mainly of streptococci [9].

ESD results in an extra-cerebral collection of suppurants located between the dura mater and the arachnoid. It is rare for the infectious process to spread directly by contiguity from a sinusitis or osteitis, gradually forming a suppurated collection which is initially extra-dural, then sub-dural and partitioned: infection of the valveless submucosal veins and sinus cavities is transmitted retrograde to the sub-dural veins. It is in this space that the infection occurs, although a meningeal reaction tends to limit it by the formation of fibrin deposits which contribute to the formation of neo-membranes and then to encapsulation [10].

The inflammatory process can spread rapidly, bilaterally and extensively, to the frontal, parietal, occipital and interhemispheric areas, given the weak links between the dura mater and the arachnoid: in 80-90% of cases, it reaches the entire supra-tentorial subdural space, especially in the frontal and parietal areas. However, extension to the base of the skull is more limited because of the close relationship between the nerve parenchyma and the base of the skull due to gravity and the presence of nerves and vessels, meaning that only 10% of ESDs are infra-tentorial[10]. This location may be secondary to direct extension following dissemination of pus from a supra-tentorial empyema, or indirect via the haematogenous route [11].

III- Epidemiological data

1. Frequency

During the period of our study we recorded 53 cases of ESDTC, i.e. 3.53 cases per year. A similar frequency was found by Kabré et al [12] who reported 30 cases of ESDTC over 9 years, i.e. 3.3 cases per year, representing 3?.03% of intracranial suppurations in the series. Elgamri et al [13] reported a lower frequency, with 16 cases of ESDTC over 9 years, or 1.8 cases per year, representing 25? % of intracranial suppurations in the series.

2. Breakdown by age

The young age of patients is found in the majority of series in the literature, especially in the second and third decades of life [16.1]. In a study carried out in 2003 in Tnde, Yend et al [18] noted a predominance of patients under 20 years of age, representing 33 to 50% of cases. In addition, an average age of between 26 and 28 years has been reported by several authors, with extremes of age ranging from 14 days to ?2 years [19]. This is probably due to the frequency of ear, nose and throat (ENT) infections at this age. In our series, the mean age was 41.5 years, with extremes of 15 and 68 years.

A breakdown by 10-year age group showed that the highest frequency was in the 15-25 age group. A similar peak in frequency was reported by Tewari et al [20] between the ages of 20 and 30 (3?%), by Nathoo et al [21] between the ages of 6 and 20 (?1%) and by Boussaad [22] between the ages of 10 and 30 (46% of cases).

3. Breakdown by gender

According to most studies, men are the most affected by CTE, particularly ESDTC, with a sex ratio varying from 2 to 5 [20,21]. Emery et al reported a sex ratio of 1.5 [23], while Kabré et al reported a sex ratio of 4.3 [12]. This predominance could be explained by socio-economic reasons, as men are more solvent and consult health facilities more easily [12]. In the Tunisian series by Kooli T et al, the sex ratio was 1.33 [24] whereas In our series, there was a clear predominance of males (sex ratio= 9.6), which is very probably related to the preponderance of males in the military population studied.

IV- Aetiological data

The aetiologies of ESDTCs vary according to the age of the patient: in infants and children, they are most often a complication of meningitis, whereas in adolescents and adults, ENT infections are the main cause [10, 20, 21].

Indeed, ENT is reported as the main cause of ESDTC by the majority of authors [10, 20, 21] and represents up to 60-90% of the causes of ETC in the literature [25]. In our series, ENT was implicated in ??.36% of cases and was the leading aetiology for ESDTC.

1- ENT cause

a- Sinusitis :

Prolonged or recurrent sinusitis is most likely to be complicated by an empyema, as inflammatory variations in the sinus mucosa encourage bone contamination and venous infection [26]. Nathoo et al [21] and Bannister et al [2?] found respectively 6?.1% and ?0% of empyemas secondary to extension of neighbouring sinusitis. This was also the case for Hilmani et al [28] and Tewari et al [20], who reported a sinus aetiology in 40% and 44.4% of cases respectively (see Table XV).

Table XV: Frequency of sinus origin by series SeriesPercentage % Sinus origin by series

BANNISTER [27]	?0
HILMANI [28]	40
NATHOO [21]	6?,1
TEWARI [20]	44,4
Our series	60.38

In our series, sinusitis was found in 60.38% of cases, dominated by frontal sinusitis and pansinusitis.

b- Otogenic origin :

The widespread use of TBAs for acute otitis media in recent decades has led to a reduction in complications such as chronic otitis media and otomastoiditis, and probably a reduction in the number of cases of CTE that could result [8]. Bannister et al [2?] reported an otogenic cause of ESDTC in 20% of cases, while Tewari et al [20] found it in 15.64% of cases. For Nathoo et al [21], it was the main cause of infra-tentorial empyema, accounting for 91% of cases [21]. In our study, otogenesis was responsible for 16.98% of ESDTCs (Table XVT).

Table XVT: Frequency of otogenic origin according to series SeriesPercentage % otogenic origin

BANNISTER [27]	20
NATHOO [21]	91
TEWARI [20]	15.6
Our series	16,98

2- Meningitis :

This infection mainly affects young children and infants, but can also be seen in adults with varying degrees of severity [10, 20, 21]. Meningitis was the 2nd most common cause of empyema in the series by Nathoo et al [21]. This origin accounted for 5.66% of the aetiologies in our patients.

3- Infection by direct seeding

This aetiology is considered to be a rare cause of ESDTC [8]. It was found in 6.5% of cases reported by Tewari et al [20]. In our study, there was one case of a neglected craniocerebral wound (1.9%).

4- Entry door unknown :

There is not always an obvious route of entry for ESDTC. In this situation, most authors agree that a haematogenous origin should be ruled out in relation to infective endocarditis, heart disease with a right/left shunt or sepsis, particularly in the context of drug addiction, as well as immunodepression, particularly by HTV, although these conditions are more likely to be complicated by cerebral abscesses than by ESDTC [10, 20, 21, 2, etc]. Cardiac ultrasound, blood cultures and HTV serology should therefore be carried out systematically whenever the route of entry is undetermined. Nathoo et al [21] found 15 patients out of 699 cases who presented with ESDTC with no known aetiology, i.e. 2% of cases, as did Hilmani et al [22]. [28] who reported only one case out of 20 of ESDTC of undetermined origin, i.e. 5% of cases. In our series, no portal of entry could be determined in 15.1% of cases, and the majority of our patients underwent cardiac ultrasound, blood cultures and HTV serology, all of which came back negative.

V-Pyogenic ESDIC in immunocompetent adults : Clinical data

The initial clinical symptomatology in ESDTC is often marked by signs of the primary disease: chronic sinusitis, chronic otitis media, meningitis, etc. A history of prior surgery or antibiotics may be responsible for an atypical clinical picture, which may delay diagnosis of the empyema and jeopardise the patient's vital prognosis [25,10]. CTE is more likely to be accompanied by fever and headache than other forms of TCA, because the brain is no longer protected by the hard meningeal membrane, and also because of the possibility of thrombosis of the veins, which are widely exposed in the subdural space. As a result, ESDTCs may be discovered when focal neurological manifestations (convulsions, focal deficits) occur in the context of a possible cerebral thrombophlebitis [8].

1- Onset and duration of symptoms

In the majority of patients in our study, i.e. 90.5% of cases, the clinical picture had developed progressively or rapidly. Brutality of symptoms was observed in 5 cases (9.4%) in patients who presented with an inaugural comititude or very frank intracranial hypertension (ICHT). A progressive onset has also been found in the majority of cases reported in the literature [10,30]. This situation could be explained by the fact that the initial clinical symptoms of ESDTC are most often masked by signs of the primary disease: chronic sinusitis, chronic otitis media, embarrure with underlying wound, meningitis. The onset is therefore difficult to pinpoint, as headache and fever can be explained by the portal of entry [10]. (Table XVTT)

Table XVTT: ESDTC installation method by series

Series	Rough	Progressive
Kabré A [12]	7 (23,3%),	23 (76,7%)
Tall [29]	1(25%)	3(75%)
Our series	5 (9,4%)	48 (90,5%)

The time taken for signs to appear can vary from a few hours to a few days [10, 21]. Emery et al [23] report a delay of between 2 and 10 days, Tewari et al [20] between 8 hours and ? days, and Jones et al [26] between 3 and 39 days. In our series, the predominance of symptoms lasting between 1 and 2 weeks was noted, with 92.45% of patients presenting with symptoms that had been evolving for less than 15 days.

2- Clinical picture

► Intracranial hypertension syndrome (ICHT) :

HTTC **is** more related to distal thrombophlebitis or even longitudinal sinus thrombophlebitis and underlying cerebral oedema than to the empyema itself, except in the case of 2: 3 mm ESDTC [10, 21]. This syndrome is present in 69 to 100% of cases [15]. Headache and vomiting are the most frequently encountered signs [12,24]. Our study found 46 patients (86.8%) who had presented with one or more signs of HTTC. These signs were found in 55% of cases reported by Emery et al [23] and in 40.6% of cases reported by Nathoo et al [21]. Papilloedema has been mentioned by some authors [10,25], but is present in only 50% of cases, which is explained by the rapid onset of HTTC in most cases. In our series, 8 patients (15%) had a fundus examination, which showed papilledema in 3 of them. This low rate may be explained by the fact that the fundus was not systematically performed in all our patients.

► Fever

The temperature is frequently 2: 38.5°C but this fever is inconstant [10, 20, 21, 23]. Fever greater than or equal to 38°C, often associated with asthenia and anorexia, was found in 39 patients, i.e. ?3.58% of cases in our series. This is in line with reports by Elgamri et al (??% of cases) [13] and Nathoo et al (??% of cases) [21]. In the series by Emery et al [23] and Alliez et al [2], fever was high, varying between 39 and 40°C in all patients.

► Meningeal signs

Tls may form part of the picture of ESDTC when the latter complicates an initial meningeal infection, and may therefore be quite marked, leading to a misdiagnosis of isolated meningitis. It is only in the presence of focal signs that a cerebral computed tomography (CT) scan is performed, revealing the presence of ESDTC [13]. In our series, these signs (stiff neck, Kernig sign, Brudzinski sign) were present in 5.66% of cases. These results differ from those of Elgamri et al [13] and Alliez et al [2], who found meningeal signs in 18%, ?% and 3?.5% of cases respectively in their series. This may well be explained by the fact that our study focused exclusively on an adult population in whom meningitis is a rare aetiology of ESDTC.

► **Focal neurological signs**

The signs revealing cerebral dysfunction result from the increase in intracranial pressure due to the accumulation of pus in the subdural space, but above all from the underlying local cerebral inflammation, thrombophlebitis of the cortical veins responsible for venous infarction and arteritis-type damage [8]. These signs are present in ?5 to 100% of patients, depending on the series [13,25]. A sensory-motor deficit was reported by Alliez et al [2] in 69% of cases, by Nathoo et al [21] in 38.5% of cases and by Loembe et al [15] in 60% of cases. In our series, they represented 26.4% of cases. Authors very often report localised or generalised comitial seizures. Emery et al [23] reported 2 cases out of 9 patients in whom epileptic seizures were noted, i.e. 22.2% of cases. For Nathoo et al [21], localised convulsions were found in 29% of cases and generalised convulsions in 4.2% of cases. In our series, they represented 22.6% of cases.Expression disorders are rarely reported by authors [13, 25]. In the series by Nathoo et al [21], only 2 patients out of 699 presented with these disorders, i.e. 0.3% of cases, whereas in the series by Hilmani [28], they were present in 25% of cases. In our study, they were present in ?.5% of patients.

► **Impaired alertness**

Disturbances of consciousness are inconstant, with a frequency ranging from 20 to 59% depending on the series [21, 23, 28]. Tls may manifest as simple obnubilation or even deep coma. Tls represented 62.5% of cases in the series by Alliez et al [2], 31.2% for Dakar et al [31] and 20% for Hilmani et al [28]. In our series they were present in ?1,?% of cases, dominated by simple somnolence. This is explained by the fact that patients with a normal neurological examination, including a good state of consciousness, are hospitalised in Tnfectiology.

► **Clinical forms**

The Bergman triad (HTTC syndrome + infectious syndrome + focal neurological signs) present in our series in 21 patients, i.e. 39.6% of cases, is the typical clinical form of ESDTC. However, the Pauci-symptomatic forms, which were the most frequent in our series (60.4% of cases), are the most prevalent in all series combined, manifested by only one or two elements of Bergman's triad [28, 31]. This triad is rarely found in the literature, reported for example in 13% of cases in Furen et al [32], 25% of cases in Yuen-hua et al [33] and 34% of cases in Pao-tsuan et al [34].

V-Para-clinical data

1. Radiological data

A new diagnostic approach has been made possible by modern imaging, spearheaded by CT scans and magnetic resonance imaging (MRI), particularly diffusion imaging. In most cases, the clinical context leads to an emergency cerebral CT scan with intravenous injection of contrast medium, which is sufficient to make the diagnosis of ESDTC [20, 21, 35].

► **Cerebral tomography**

Cerebral CT reveals a highly characteristic lesion consisting of a hypodense subdural extra-axial collection with peripheral contrast, which may be associated with peri-lesional vasogenic oedema (Figure 5, 6). However, it can be extremely difficult to distinguish a chronic subdural haematoma in the absence of any infectious context [30, 31]. It also allows the location, number and type of suppurations to be determined, and the impact on the surrounding cerebral parenchyma to be assessed [8]. In our study, this characteristic lesion was found in 98.11% of cases and vasogenic cerebral oedema was associated with ESDTC in 15.1% of cases. In the series by Coulibaly et al [36], this characteristic lesion was found in 81.48% of patients and cerebral oedema was associated with ESDTC in 44.4% of cases. Similarly, in the series by Kabré et al [12], cerebral CT showed a typical image in 2? cases (90%).

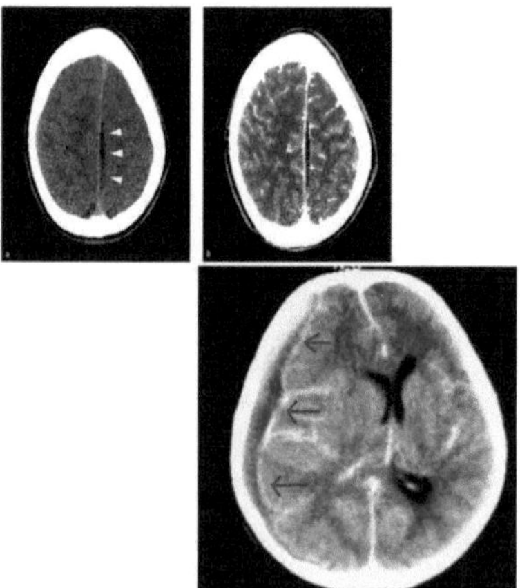

Figure 5: CT scan of ESDIC (left interhemispheric location) a: SPC; b: APC

Figure 6: Right hemispheric ESDTC (CT brain-APC)

ESDTC is most often a single lesion, but multiple and bilateral locations are not uncommon [21] (Figure 6, ?). In our study, the lesion was single in 94.3% of cases, multiple in 5.5% of cases and of variable thickness, ranging from approximately 1mm to 08mm (Table XVTTT). These results are comparable to those reported by Zimmerman et al who found a single lesion in 90% of cases [38] and Coulibaly et al [36] who found that the lesion was single in 80% of cases and multiple in 20% of cases [36]. The lesion was also single in ?0% of cases reported by Hilmani [28] and multiple localisation was noted in the study by Fuerman et al [39] and in that by Nathoo et al [21] in 33.3% and 15% of cases respectively.

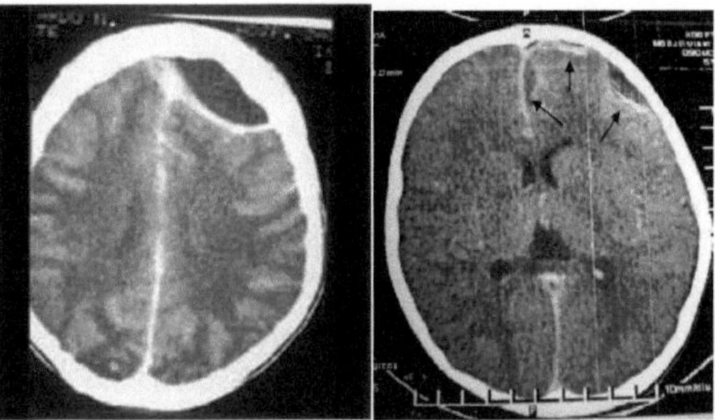

Figure 7: Frontal ESD

Figure 8: Multiple ESD

(Cerebral CT-APC) (Cerebral CT-APC) (Cerebral CT -APC) (Cerebral CT-APC) APC)

Table XVIII: Number of ESDICs by series SeriesSingle lesionMultiple lesions

Zimmerman [38]	90%	10%
Coulibaly [36]	80%	20%
Hilmani [28]	?0%	30%
Fuerman [39]	66,?%	33.3%
Nathoo [21]	85%	15%
Our series	94.3%	5.?%

The authors report that there is no relationship between the portal of entry and the site of the ETC [36], although Jones et al [26] reported that the The most common location for ESDTC secondary to rhinosinusitis was in the frontal region. ESDTC is most frequently found in the convex region, especially in the frontal region in 80% of cases and in the interhemispheric region in 12% of cases [18, 40]. In our series, the preferred site was supratentorial (98% of cases) and the posterior cerebral fossa (Figure 8) was involved in only 1 case (1.9%). The most frequent location was frontal (35.85% of cases) and hemispheric collections (Figure 9, 10) accounted for 20.5% of cases. These results are comparable to those of BOK et al [41] who reported a convex location in 68.8% of cases, with 34% of cases found in the fronto-parietal region and 3% of cases in the inter-hemispheric region (Table XTX).

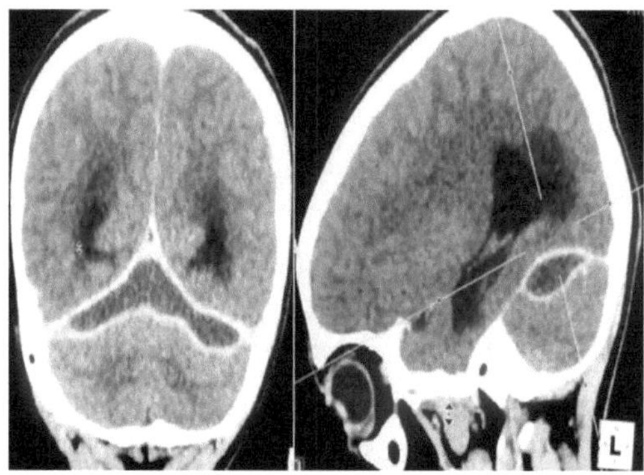

Figure 9: ESDTC of the posterior cerebral fossa (CT brain-APC)

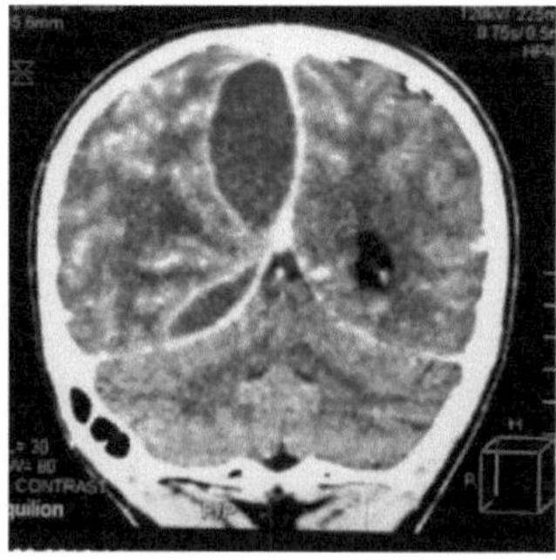

Figure 10: Inter-hemispheric ESDTC (CT brain-APC)

Similarly, Nathoo et al [21] reported that 51.8% of ESDTCs in their series were located in the convexity, 20.9% of cases in the interhemisphere, with a combination of these two locations in 2?.5% of cases, and subtentorial location was noted in only 2.6% of cases. Similarly, according to Ouiminga et al, the preferred location was supra-tentorial in 89% of cases, of which 35% were frontal, 24% parietal and 10% inter-hemispheric. Only one case was located in the posterior cerebral fossa.

Table XIX: ESDIC locations by series

Series Number **of cases**

Convexity Inter- hemispheric FCP

BOK [41]	90	62 (68,8%)	34 (37%)	4 (4,4%)
Nathoo [21]	699	362 (51,8%)	146 (20,9)	18 (2,6%)
HILMAN I [28]	20	12(60%)	3(15%)	2(10%)
Our series	53	19 (35,85%)	4 (7,55%)	1 (1,9%)

Cerebral CT can also be used to diagnose associated lesions (intra-parenchymal abscesses, extra-dural empyema), complications (sinus thrombosis, cerebral involvement) and to suspect a possible portal of entry (sinusitis, meningitis, osteitis) [40]. In our study, an associated abscess was found in one patient, and sinus filling indicating sinusitis or pansinusitis was noted in 32 patients. Subfalcoral involvement was found in 36 patients.

► **Cerebral magnetic resonance imaging (MRI) with diffusion sequences**

MRT is a diagnostic tool that complements CT perfectly in terms of cerebral infections, and the advent of diffusion sequences in particular, and to a lesser extent spectroscopy and perfusion sequences, has enabled the radiologist to play a full part in the positive diagnosis of infection, particularly in the case of ESDTC with pyogenic germs, thus making it possible to eliminate lesions whose scannographic or even para-magnetic behaviour could be similar to them, to dissociate extra- and sub-dural collections and, above all, to detect small lesions [42, 43].

It has been reported by several authors to be the examination of choice for the diagnosis and monitoring of ESDTCs, especially those located in the temporal fossa, sub-temporal and sub-frontal base, and in the PCF [20, 21, 23, 44]. This is because any artefacts due to bone, which are particularly troublesome on CT, are absent, the delineation of the different elements (bone, CSF, parenchyma) is more precise, contrast enhancement allows better localisation, and the contribution of diffusion sequences and, to a lesser extent, spectroscopy also allows better characterisation of the nature of the effusion (blood, sterile effusion or pus) [45]. Similarly, MRT provides better evidence of cerebral oedema and ischaemic lesions, and angio-MRT is also effective in detecting associated sinus thrombosis [45].

For example, pyogenic ESDTCs may be difficult to detect on CT due to their proximity to the bony vault, especially if the collection is small. However, their behaviour on MRT is similar to that of pyogenic brain abscesses: subdural collection frankly hypointense on T1, hyperintense on T2 and on FLATR, associated or not with an intraparenchymal digitiform FLATR hypersignal corresponding to cerebral oedema, with peripheral enhancement of the collection on gadolinium injection corresponding to the shell (Figure 10). On diffusion imaging, these collections are hyperintense with a reduction in the apparent diffusion coefficient (ADC) on the ADC map, which in almost all cases makes it possible to distinguish between an ESDTC and a chronic subdural haematoma or a CSF hygroma [42, 44] (Figure 11).

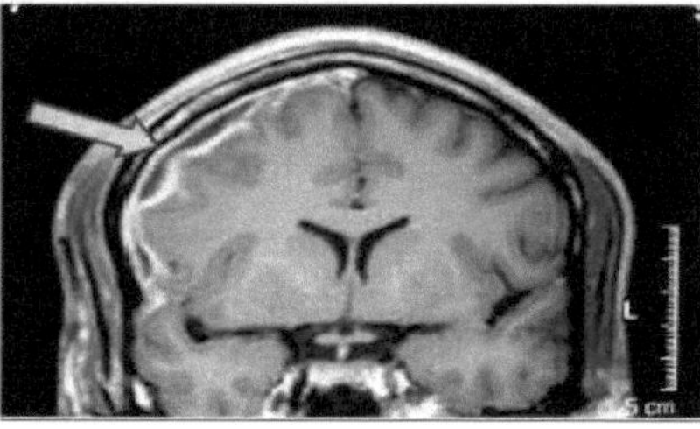

Figure 11: Right fronto-temporal ESDTC on morphological MRT (T1 Gado)

DWI ADC

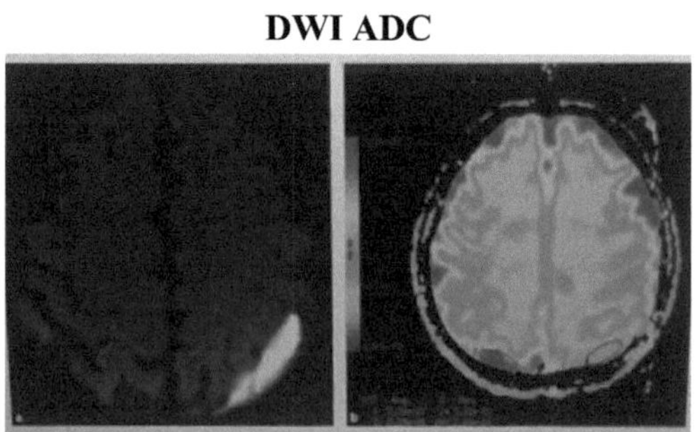

Figure 12: Aspect of ESDTC on diffusion MRT

Spectroscopy could also show the presence of an amino acid peak centred at 0.9 ppm in the subdural collection, confirming the purulent nature of the subdural collection, but its absence does not rule out the diagnosis. The presence of associated peaks of succinate, acetate and lactate would also be highly suggestive but non-specific [44]. Perfusion MRT has no place in the diagnosis of ESDTC [44]. Cerebral MRT was performed in only one patient in our series (1.9% of cases). None of the patients underwent spectroscopy or perfusion sequences.

2. Biological data

The biological inflammatory syndrome, with elevated SV and CRP, is frequently found in pyogenic ESDTC, but is inconsistent. Similarly, hyperleukocytosis with a predominance of neutrophils, although frequent, may also be absent, particularly in cases of prior antibiotic treatment [44,45]. A predominantly neutrophilic hyperleukocytosis was present in 60 to ?4.1% of patients in the series by Yuen-hua et al [33], the series by Furen et al [32] and Coulibaly et al [36]. Hyperleukocytosis was present in 58.5% of our patients with an accelerated sedimentation rate in 41.5 of cases. CRP, performed in 3? patients, was elevated in 51.35% of cases.

3. Bacteriological data

The bacteriological study of subdural pus samples depends on the conditions under which the pus is collected in the operating theatre, the short time taken for culture in the laboratory and the use of multiple culture media. Optimum conditions for isolating the germ therefore require close collaboration between the neurosurgeon, the laboratory technician and the bacteriologist [20, 21, 40, 46]. When all the steps, from collecting the pus in the operating theatre to culturing it in the various media in the laboratory, are carried out carefully and meticulously, the chance of isolating the causative germ approaches 100% in some series [46,4?] It is recommended to inoculate abscess pus directly into aerobic (1ml), anaerobic (1ml), Lowenstein and Sabouraud blood culture bottles during the operation. From a practical point of view, it is sufficient to inoculate the blood culture bottles and keep the rest of the pus in a sterile bottle at room temperature so that it can be inoculated as soon as possible in the laboratory on specialised media, when the empyema is evacuated. done outside normal working hours. In this respect, it is essential for surgeons to be trained to take bacteriological samples under good conditions [46, 4...].

In the earliest studies, the germ most frequently encountered was Staphylococcus aureus. Today, more than 50% of cases are sterile pus, and some are polymicrobial. The germs most frequently reported today are Streptococci, Staphylococci, anaerobic germs and Gram(-) bacilli [4?]. The bacteriological study of the empyema pus was carried out in the 48 cases operated on in our department. The pathogen was found in only 3 cases, i.e. 6.25% of the samples taken. The germs found in our series were :

- Streptococcus milleri (aerobic, gram-positive cocci, sinus origin): 1 case
- Streptococcus sp (aerobic, gram+ cocci, origin unknown): 1 case
- Brevibacterium spp (aerobic, gram-positive bacillus, otogenic origin): 1 case

The sample was sterile in 45 cases, i.e. 93.5% of samples taken.

For Kabré et al [12] and Coulibaly et al [36], the bacteriological study of the pus sample was sterile in almost 90% of cases. For Tewari et al [20] and Leys et al [10], culture was also negative in ?0% and 50% of cases respectively. However, for Jones et al [26], the germ was found in almost 90% of cases. The germs reported by these authors were essentially Streptococcus and Staphylococcus [10, 12, 20, 26, 36].

There is therefore considerable variability in the results of culture of empyema pus between the different series described in the literature, and this is due either to poor technique in the methods of collection, transport or culture of the pus, or to the prior introduction of antibiotic therapy pre-operatively.

Furthermore, concordance between the germ isolated from the portal of entry and that isolated from the empyema pus is not always constant [20]. Kaufman et al [48] noted discordance in ?5% of cases, while Hilmani [28] et al reported concordance in 100% of cases. In our series, culture of the auricular pus was carried out in 8 patients, and came back sterile each time.

Finally, it should be noted that lumbar puncture is contraindicated in the presence of signs of intracranial hypertension or focal neurological signs, even in the presence of meningeal signs in the foreground, if emergency cerebral neuroimaging has not ruled out a large intra- or extra-axial intracranial expansive lesion [120]. When it is carried out, it often shows a germ-free cellular reaction [49]. Kaufmann et al [48] even reported 4 cases with signs of cerebral involvement within 6 hours of LP. Performed on 3 patients in our series (before they were referred to us), it showed purulent CSF with no germs on direct examination or culture in all 3 cases.

VI- Therapeutic methods

ESDTCs are potentially serious injuries requiring urgent treatment [20,21]. Conventional treatment has always involved urgent surgical evacuation combined with antibiotic therapy, but the choice of surgical technique (hole evacuation or craniotomy) has until recently been the subject of controversy [41]. In addition, experience of exclusive medical treatment for small brain abscesses (:S 3 cm) and the advent of new generations of TBAs has made it possible to envisage exclusive medical treatment for pyogenic ESDTC without significant neurological repercussions, based on the results of bacteriological samples and combined with treatment of the entry site, for a period of up to 3 months in certain extreme cases [20, 21, 41, 44]. However, surgery should be performed if there are signs of HTTC, focal neurological signs or if the ESDTC increases in volume under treatment [50]. After evacuation of the collection, drainage for a few days has often been recommended by authors [51]. In our series, exclusive medical treatment was instituted in 9.4% of cases and medical-surgical treatment was undertaken in 90.6% of cases, with a combination of medical treatment / trepanation in 84.94% of cases and medical treatment / craniotomy in 5.66% of cases. (5,66%).

1. Medical treatment

Once the diagnosis has been confirmed, medical treatment must be started: this is based on broad-spectrum antibiotic therapy, with or without anti-oedematous agents and sometimes anti-convulsants.

► Antibiotic therapy

Broad-spectrum antibiotic therapy should be started as soon as possible, by parenteral route, immediately after taking bacteriological samples (pus, blood cultures, ear swabs), on which the choice of different molecules will subsequently depend. It should be based on a combination of bactericidal antibiotics capable of crossing the blood-brain and blood-meningeal barriers [44]. If the causative germ is isolated and an antibiotic susceptibility test is available, antibiotic therapy should be adapted according to the different antibiotic sensitivities [20, 21, 44]. If cultures are negative, then broad-spectrum antibiotic therapy should be maintained, to cover the various possible germs depending on the likely route of entry, and to act on both aerobic and anaerobic germs, given the frequency of their concomitance [20, 21, 44, 51].

It is therefore currently recommended to combine at least one 3ème generation cephalosporin with a nitroimidazole [51]. The combination of cefotaxime (Claforan®) + metronidazole (Flagyl®) appears to be the most frequently used in the literature, due to its availability, cost and, above all, efficacy, particularly in cases of ENT aetiology of ESDTC [51]. Fosfomycin (Fosfocine®), vancomycin (Vancocine®) or rifampicin (Rifadine®) may be added if Staphylococcus is suspected, as well as ciprofloxacin (Cipro500 ®) if Pseudomonas is suspected [51] (Table XX). There is also no consensus on the total duration of antibiotic therapy [51]. However, the majority of authors agree that the minimum duration of intravenous antibiotic therapy is 4 weeks in the case of medical-surgical treatment, and 6 weeks in the case of exclusive medical treatment [51]. There has also been no consensus on oral retreatment [51].

Table XX: Recommended TBA combinations for pyogenic ESDIC

sinus origin	Otogenic origin	Origin unknown	Origin post-traumatic
Cefotaxime 12glj +	Cefotaxime 12glj +	Cefotaxime 12glj +	Cefotaxime 12glj +
Metronidazole 1, glj	Metronidazole 1, glj +l-	Metronidazole 1, glj	Metronidazole 1, glj +
	Ciprofloxacin 1,2glj	+l- Fosfomycin 12glj or Vancomycin 2glj	Fosomycin 12glj or Vancomycin 2glj
	(because Pseudomonas possible)	(because Staphylococcus possible)	(because Staphylococcus is common)

The combination of cefotaxime, fosfomycin and metronidazole was used most frequently in our series (69.8%). The average duration of parenteral treatment was 34.5 days, with a minimum of 22 days and a maximum of 4? days. It should be noted that 6 patients in our series benefited from oral relay: ciprofloxacin in 4 cases and rifampicin + ciprofloxacin in 2 cases. All other authors have also used a probabilistic combination of parenteral broad-spectrum TBAs for a period of 4 to 8 weeks, and then adapted to the results of the antibiogram in the event of a positive bacteriological sample [20, 21, 2?, 40, 41, 44, 51, 52].

► **Other treatments**

The cerebral oedema that may accompany ESDTC may give rise to a HTTC syndrome, and anti-oedematous treatment should therefore be instituted when there are clear clinical and/or radiological signs of HTTC, especially in the acute phase [53]. Furthermore, seizures are frequent in supra-tentorial locations of ESDTC, given the associated venous infarcts, hence the recommendation by some authors to systematically institute prophylactic anti-coma treatment in all patients with supra-tentorial empyema, which should be maintained for 18 to 24 months, with a minimum of 6 months [53]. Our series included ? patients who had presented with cerebral oedema, i.e. 13.21% of cases, which led to their being put on dexamethasone at a dose of 8 to 12 mg/d, for a period of 3 to 8 days. As for comitiality, 12 patients (22.6%) had suffered a convulsive seizure, and all were treated with anti-convulsants.

2. Surgical treatment

Surgery is required if the volume of the empyema shows signs of HTTC or if it increases in size under treatment. There is no real correlation between the initial thickness of the ESDTC and the surgical decision, but most authors agree that evacuation is necessary in the case of a hemispherical ESD thicker than 3mm, especially as the mass effect on the medial structures is significant and the subject is young [20, 21, 40, 41, 44, 51]. Tl may be limited to 1, 2 or even 3 trepan holes, which can be enlarged as desired by means of a craniectomy with durotomies opposite the subdural collection, or require a large craniotomy flap with durotomy, allowing complete evacuation of the empyema and wide excision of the outer wall of its shell [41, 44]. The timing of the operation is just as important as the surgical technique, and the speed with which the diagnosis is made and surgical treatment initiated, as well as effective treatment of the portal of entry, are generally far more important than the choice of surgical technique [20, 21, 44]. According to the majority of authors, only subtentorial subdural empyema, which has a very serious course, should be treated by wide craniectomy or craniotomy [20, 21, 23, 44], although some rare authors prefer trepanation [54]. Post-operative subdural or subcutaneous drainage is optional and depends essentially on the habits of each team [20, 21, 52, 54, 55]. In our series, 90.6% of patients received surgical treatment combined with ATB. Practically the same percentage was reported by Coulibaly et al [36] (85.18%), Elgamri et al [13] (81%), Kooli et al [24] and others. (95%), Nathoo et al (96%) and Tewari et al [20] (9?%).

► **Trepanning**

Since the end of the 19th century, there has been an abundance of work devoted to Neolithic cranial trepanations. At the source, the discoveries made by Dr Prunières on the Grands Causses in Gévaudan in 18?0 revealed the very first trepanations identified as such, some of which date back to the Vth millennium BC. [56]. A simple trephine hole, enlarged by a craniectomy or trephine washer, this technique has been used by the majority of authors. It consists of evacuating the pus from the ESD through a simple hole or a small bone washer, after performing a small durotomy to gain access to the subdural space. Some people even prefer to make 2 or 3 holes, although this has not really been shown to be superior in various studies [21, 41, 54]. The cavity is then washed with warm saline and subdural or subcutaneous drainage for 48 hours is inserted as an option [5?] (Figure 12).

A b

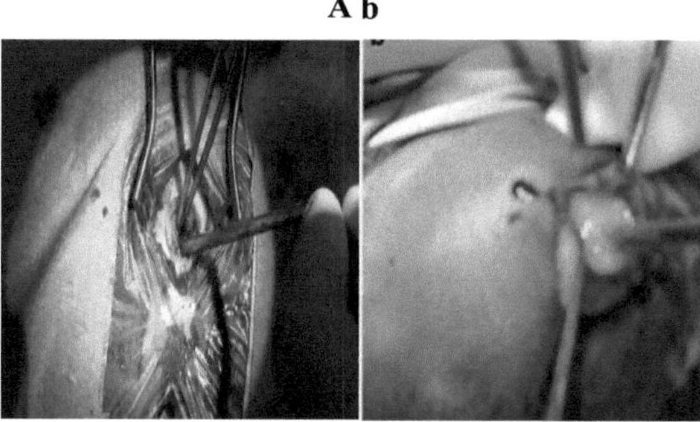

Figure 13: Removal of ESD by trepanation; a: drilling of the bone hole / b: evacuation of pus after durotomy

However, wide craniectomy is better indicated as 1st-line treatment for evacuation of ESDTCs from the posterior cerebral fossa, given the anatomical features and small size of this area, as well as the frequency of cerebellar oedema often associated with the risk of tonsillar involvement [20, 41, 44, 48, 54, 58], but trepanation is still possible even in this location [54]. However, for some authors, this technique offers insufficient exposure of the subdural space, which could even be poorly centred in relation to the collection in the event of poor positioning by the surgeon, with difficulty in evacuation in the event of thick pus or a thick or multi-partitioned shell, which could lead to insufficient evacuation of ESDTC and be a source of recurrence [21]. However, no study to date has shown that craniotomy is superior to trepanation for the evacuation of ESDTC, or that trepanation is associated with a higher rate of recurrence or morbidity in general [20, 41, 44, 48, 54, 58]. This technique was used in ?8% of cases by Bok et al [41], 89% of cases by Tewari et al [20], 8?.8% of cases by Coulibaly et al [36] and ?9% of cases by Ouiminga et al [40]. In our series, 36 patients (6?.92%) underwent 2-hole trepanation, 3 patients underwent single-hole trepanation and 6 patients underwent craniectomy to enlarge the hole(s), for a total of 84.94% trepanation/craniectomy surgery.

► Craniotomy

It consists of creating a bone flap opposite the collection in order to gain direct access to the collection by means of a wide durotomy, to be able to excise the outer wall of the shell and evacuate the pus in addition to abundant washing with warm saline, and then to replace the bone flap with optional subdural or subcutaneous drainage [21, 5?]. For some authors, such as Nathoo et al [21] and Bannister et al [2?], this remains the surgical technique of choice for the evacuation of ESDTC, although to date there is no evidence that it is superior to trepanation, especially as it requires a much larger skin incision with a greater risk of intra-operative blood spoliation and post-operative acute subdural or extra-dural haematomas. [20, 41, 44, 48, 54, 58].

A b

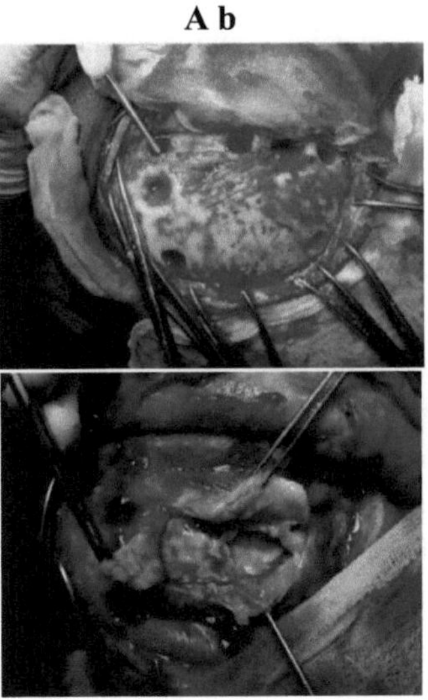

Figure 14: Evacuation of ESDTC by craniotomy; a: Carrying out the craniotomy; b: Wide durotomy with excision of the external wall of the shell and evacuation of the pus.

In our series, 3 patients (5.66%) underwent craniotomy to evacuate the empyema: this was necessary in 2ème 2 patients after initial evacuation by trepanation, and was the first choice in only one patient when extremely dense pus could not be evacuated through the trepan holes.

► Treatment of the front door :

Treatment of the entry site is essential to avoid relapses and minimise recurrences [54, 55]. This may involve medical treatment or, more often, a medico-surgical treatment combining an additional procedure such as drainage of a pathological sinus or petro-mastoid evisceration, carried out either at the same time as evacuation of the ESD or at a later date [20, 44, 55]. In our series, 36 patients out of 53, i.e. 6?.92% of cases, were able to benefit from curative treatment of the portal of entry, which was ENT in the vast majority of cases, in line with most authors whose rates of treatment of the portal of entry in their patients varied from 61 to ??% according to the different series studied [20, 21, 41, 44, 48, 54, 58].

► Monitoring during treatment

The medical or medico-surgical management of pyogenic ESDTC is inconceivable without rigorous monitoring throughout hospitalisation, in order to assess efficacy and adapt subsequent therapeutic decisions (change of TBA, repeat surgery), and to detect possible adverse effects of treatment or the occurrence of complications, especially in the case of exclusive medical treatment [13, 20, 21, 44]. Monitoring should be both clinical (regression of HTTC signs, improvement in focal neurological signs, thermal defervescence) and biological (lowering of the SV and CRP, normalisation of the leucocyte count and absence of haematopoietic repercussions of ATB on the CBC or ionic repercussions on the blood ionogram, absence of repercussions of ATBs on renal function) and neuroradiological (reduction in the size of the ESD, regression of cerebral oedema, reduction in the mass effect on medial structures, clearing of sinus or oto-mastoid cavities). For this reason, a daily clinical examination combined with a bi-weekly biological check-up and a cerebral CT scan without and with injection of iodinated contrast product carried out within 24 to 48 hours post-operatively and then every two weeks thereafter are essential. ? to 10 days until the end of treatment (or as an emergency in the event of the slightest deterioration in neurological condition) would seem to represent a more than satisfactory regimen. satisfactory monitoring of treatment [13, 20,

21, 33, 34, 36, 41, 44, 51, 52, 58, 59].

VII- Complications

► Brain engagement :

Not specific to ESDTC, cerebral involvement can complicate any intracranial neoventric volume [44]. Subfalcrial involvement is the most common but does not always manifest itself clinically, and clinical manifestations lack specificity, although it is indicative of increased intracranial pressure. Temporal involvement is usually manifested by homolateral anisocoria associated with hemiparesis, or even contralateral heminecerebration, but the mere presence of pupillary asymmetry is enough to suggest the diagnosis. Cerebellar involvement is classically manifested by the appearance of frank stiffness of the neck progressing to generalised hypertonic or even opisthotonic seizures, associated with neurovegetative disorders, particularly respiratory, and the appearance of the slightest of these signs in a patient presenting with ESD of the posterior cerebral fossa should raise fears of the occurrence of this complication [44]. Of course, if there is cerebral involvement, the ESDTC must be evacuated immediately [21, 40, 44]. In our study, we found mainly radiological subfalcial involvement (6?,9% of cases) but also two cases of temporal involvement (3?,?% of cases).

► Cerebral venous thrombosis :

This is a rare complication, affecting the venous dural sinuses more than the cerebral cortical veins, and mainly involving the superior sagittal sinus for supratentorial ESDTC and the sigmoid and transverse sinuses for subtentorial ESDTC (generally related to mastoiditis) [44, 54, 55]. It may be asymptomatic and its clinical manifestations are non-specific, consisting of a progressive increase in signs of intracranial hypertension, which may lead to coma. The diagnosis is confirmed by CT scan, but especially by cerebral MRI, which shows a an intra-luminal gap in a dural sinus (empty delta sign) and a lack of opacification downstream of the thrombosis, particularly on the cerebral phlebogram, which may be associated with cerebral turgidity and/or cerebellar turgidity in the most advanced cases [55]. Treatment is based on curative doses of heparin therapy, combined with antibiotic therapy and treatment of the possible oto-mastoid portal of entry, but the outcome remains uncertain [55]. In our series, two patients presented with sinus venous thrombosis (3.8%), including one case of thrombosis of the superior sagittal sinus and one case of thrombosis of the left sigmoid sinus.

► **Comitology:**

Although it is frequently part of the inaugural clinical picture of ESDTC (already described in the clinical signs), it nevertheless represents a complication due to cortical irritation [21,44]. The treatment of convulsive seizures is based on the direct intravenous administration of benzodiazepines (in particular Clonazepam: Rivotril®), but the management of comitiality associated with ESDTCs is based above all on prophylactic anti-comitial treatment, which should be implemented systematically in the event of convulsive seizures, or even in the event of any supratentorial localisation, according to certain authors [21, 44, 4?], given the high risk of secondary convulsions (25 to 50% of cases) [21, 44, 4?]. In our series, comitology was found in 22.6% of cases.

VIII- Course and prognosis

► **Evolution :**

The outcome is all the more favourable, with maximum or even complete neurological recovery, when the treatment of pyogenic ESDTC is rapidly implemented and bacteriologically appropriate [44, 60, 61]. Tewari et al [20] reported a favourable outcome in ??.8% of cases, as did 82% of cases in the series by Nathoo et al [21], 85% of cases in the series by Coulibaly et al [36], 86% of cases in the series by Bok et al [41] and 62.5% of cases in the series by Emery et al [23]. In our series, 50 patients (94.34%) had a favourable outcome. At the On leaving the neurosurgery department, they were all independent and able to carry out normal daily activities. However, the mortality associated with ESDTC, even with well-managed treatment, remains significant according to the different series, varying from 4.4 to 12.2% of cases, which testifies to the potential seriousness of this pathology despite the progress made in neuroradiology and broad-spectrum antibiotic therapy [20, 21, 24, 2?, 41, 44, 4?, 62] . In our series, 3 patients (5.66%) died, including one case of septic shock on post-op day 2, one case of brain death with neurovegetative disorders on post-op day 3 and one case of massive pulmonary embolism on post-op day 9.

► **Prognostic factors linked to progression :**

Many prognostic factors vary from one series to another, and this is most likely due to the particularities of the different groups of patients studied in each case.

For Nathoo et al [21], for example, evacuation of the ESDTC by means of a craniotomy, as well as the supratentorial location of the ESD, were significantly associated with a favourable outcome, unlike Bok et al [22]. [41] in which the latter was significantly related to evacuation of the ESDTC by simple trepanation. As for Tewari et al [20] and Hlavin et al [62], none of the above factors was important for prognosis but it was reported that the duration of symptoms was significantly inversely related to favourable outcome. However, the only prognostic factor significantly associated with outcome found in most of the series studied [13, 20, 21, 24, 2?, 36, 40, 41, 44, 4?, 62] was the state of consciousness on admission, assessed objectively by the Glasgow score (GCS). A normal or slightly altered state of consciousness on admission (GCS 2: 12/15) was significantly associated with a favourable outcome, while an altered state of consciousness on admission (GCS < 12/15) was significantly associated with an unfavourable outcome, and would generally indicate complicated forms of ESDTC.In our series, age, sex, duration of symptoms, site of PDS, route of onset and treatment modalities showed no relationship with patient outcome. The only statistically significant prognostic factor identified was the initial state of consciousness ($p < 0.01$), in line with the results described in the literature.

► **Long-term follow-up and prognosis :**

Patients treated for pyogenic ESDTC should receive regular follow-up at the neurosurgery outpatient clinic, based on clinical examination and cerebral CT scan without and with injection of iodinated contrast. There is no consensus in the literature regarding the frequency of CT scan monitoring after the end of treatment, but it is accepted that at least one cerebral CT scan (or MRT) without and with injection of contrast medium should be performed within one month of the end of treatment, since recurrences of pyogenic ESDTC are exceptional in properly treated immunocompetent adults, and virtually all occur in individuals who are either immunocompromised or who have not had adequate treatment of the portal of entry, something which is extremely important to check during the various consultations. The complete disappearance of the empyema or its replacement by CSF, particularly in hemispheric ESDTCs in older subjects, and the disappearance of peripheral contrast should be sought [20, 21, 44, 62]. In addition, motor deficits and comititude dominate the conditions encountered during follow-up in the various publications studied [13, 20, 21, 36, 40, 44, 4?] Patients with motor deficits should therefore be referred to a functional rehabilitation centre, or even an occupational therapy centre for those most affected. Similarly, all patients treated for ESDTC who have developed comititude should systematically receive anti-epileptic treatment, which should be continued for at least 18 to 24 months, and some authors even recommend systematic prophylaxis for any supratentorial location of ESDTC, given the high risk of comititude [21, 44, 4?, 53]. Of the 50 living patients discharged, 4 were lost to follow-up. The other patients all underwent a follow-up brain CT scan with or without PDC injection within a month of discharge. Thus, 91.30% of patients had 2 consultations and 2 follow-up brain CT scans in the 3 months following discharge. Anti-epileptic treatment was maintained for at least 1 year in ?5% of patients who developed comititude. There was no recurrence in any patient. Assessment of quality of life is therefore an important aspect of follow-up for ESDTC. This assessment is not easy, as it will have to take account of motor, sensory and sensory deficits, motor rehabilitation and socio-professional reintegration in patients who have been treated [44, 21, 62].

CONCLUSIONS

Intracranial empyema accounts for 31% to 65% of intracranial suppurations, depending on the series published. Subdural empyema is the most common site and is most often associated with a pyogenic infection. They represent a genuine medical and surgical emergency.

Intracranial subdural empyemas are purulent collections that develop in the subdural space. Their management has been profoundly modified by advances in modern neuroimaging. Treatment is essentially based on broad-spectrum antibiotic therapy, with or without surgery. However, there is no consensus on the best therapeutic approach.

In our work, we studied the management of intracranial subdural empyema by the neurosurgery department of the Military Hospital of Tunis concerning 53 patients over a period of 15 years (January 2000 to December 2014), in order to propose a standardised management of intracranial subdural empyema with pyogenic germs in immunocompetent adults. Intracranial subdural empyemas of tuberculous, fungal, parasitic or postoperative origin, occurring in children and immunocompromised patients, as well as extra-dural empyemas and cerebral abscesses, were excluded from our study.

We studied the epidemiological, aetiological, clinical and radiological data, the contribution of complementary examinations, the different therapeutic attitudes, the means of monitoring and the evolutionary consequences after 2 years, and compared our results with those of other published series. In our series, we found an annual frequency of 3.53 cases per year, with an average age of 41.5 years and a predominance of males, with a sex ratio of 9.6. The aetiologies found were dominated by locoregional infection, mainly ENT, in 83% of cases, including sinusitis, especially frontal sinusitis (60.38%), and oto-mastoiditis (16.98%). The portal of entry was not found in 15.1% of cases.

The clinical signs most frequently found were intracranial hypertension syndrome in 86.8% of cases, infectious syndrome in ?3.58% of cases and focal neurological signs in 45.28% of cases, dominated by motor deficits (26.41%) and convulsions (22.6%). The classic Bergman triad, representing the typical clinical form, was present in only 39.6% of cases, while the pauci-symptomatic clinical forms were the most frequent (60.4% of cases).

A 1st-line cerebral CT scan without and with injection of contrast medium was performed in all patients. This alone allowed the diagnosis of cerebral empyema in 98.11% of cases. Cerebral MRT with gadolinium injection and diffusion sequence was performed in one patient (1.9%). This confirmed the diagnosis of subdural empyema suspected on the CT scan.

The neuroradiological examinations showed a predominance of supratentorial localisations (98.1% of cases), as well as single localisations (94.3% of cases). The most frequent locations were frontal (35.85% of cases) and hemispheric (20.0% of cases).The pathogen was found in only 3 cases, or 6.25% of the samples taken. In 45 cases (93.5%), the sample was sterile. In our series, only bacteriological study of the empyema pus enabled the pathogen to be identified. Samples taken from the portal of entry and lumbar punctures were sterile on each occasion. The germs found in our series were Streptococcus milleri (1 case), Streptococcus sp (1 case) and Brevibacterium spp (1 case). Biological tests showed hyperleukocytosis on the NFS in 58.5% of cases, an accelerated VS in 41.5% of cases and an elevated CRP in 51.35% of cases. Treatment was exclusively medical in 9.4% of cases and surgical in 90.6%.
Medical treatment was based on a combination of parenteral broad-spectrum antibiotics in all patients. The most commonly used combination was Cefotaxime/Fosfomycin/Metronidazole in 69.8% of cases, for a mean duration of 34.5 days. Treatment of cerebral oedema with corticosteroids was associated with antibiotic therapy in 13.21% of cases, and anti-epileptic treatment was used in 22.6% of cases. Surgical treatment consisted of trepanation in 84.94% of cases (2-hole in 6?.92% of cases, single-hole in 5.66% of cases and extended by craniectomy in 11.32% of cases) and craniotomy in 5.66% of cases.

Treatment of the portal of entry, when identified, was carried out in 6?.92% of cases.As regards monitoring during treatment, all patients underwent daily clinical monitoring, with at least a bi-weekly CBC with or without SV and/or CRP in 96.24% of cases.Cerebral CT was the most important means of neuro-radiological monitoring: 91.66% of patients had a follow-up cerebral CT scan without and with contrast injection within 24 to 48 hours of empyema evacuation. Non-operated patients and those stable post-operatively had a follow-up cerebral CT scan every ? to 10 days in ?1,?% of cases.

In 96.2% of cases, the follow-up cerebral CT scan performed during the last week of hospitalisation showed: a significant reduction in the thickness of the subdural collection (:S 2mm), a clear regression or even disappearance of the cerebral oedema opposite, a reduction in peripheral contrast, and even the absence of a subdural collection.The most frequent complications were brain damage (?1,?%) and comitial seizures (22.6%).On discharge, 94.34% of patients had a favourable outcome and 5.66% an unfavourable outcome (3 patients died).

The only prognostic factor significantly related to outcome that we were able to identify was the state of consciousness on admission. A Glasgow score < 12/15 on admission was significantly associated with an unfavourable outcome, and a

Glasgow score 2: 12/15 on admission was significantly associated with a favourable outcome, with $p < 0.01$.

During follow-up of patients at the neurosurgery outpatient clinic, over a period of 2 years, 4 patients were lost to follow-up and 91.3% of the remaining patients received at least 2 consultations and 2 follow-up brain CT scans without and with contrast injection in the 3 months following discharge.

Among these 46 patients, no recurrence of the empyema was noted; 22 patients, or 44% of cases, showed complete normalisation of the cerebral CT at 1[er] scan control; 2 patients (4%) who had never convulsed presented with comitiality. Anti-epileptic treatment was maintained for at least 1 year in ?5% of patients who had already convulsed during hospitalisation.

We can therefore conclude from the various data studied in the literature, as well as from our own series, that pyogenic subdural empyema in immunocompetent adults is still a topical condition in various countries, whatever their degree of development, and that its management must be multidisciplinary.

The main cause is the spread of locoregional infections, particularly oto-sinus infections. The typical clinical form of intracranial subdural empyema is rarely present and the clinical picture can sometimes mislead the diagnosis.

The CBC, VS and CRP can guide the diagnosis in frustrated forms, but are frequently normal.Cerebral CT without and with injection of contrast medium is the key examination, enabling the diagnosis to be made in the majority of cases. Cerebral diffusion MRI is an essential adjunct to the diagnosis in cases where the distinction between intracranial subdural empyema and other differential diagnoses, particularly chronic subdural haematoma, may be difficult or impossible. Lumbar puncture has no place in the bacteriological diagnosis of subdural empyema, and in some cases is even contraindicated because of the risk of iatrogenic cerebral involvement. Bacteriological diagnosis is essentially based on isolation of the germ from the empyema pus. However, poor sample conditioning and inoculation techniques in the various culture media are responsible for a large number of sterile cultures. The germs most often implicated are essentially Streptococci and Staphylococci, followed by anaerobes and Gram (-) bacilli.The medical treatment of subdural intracranial empyema caused by pyogenic germs is essentially based on a probabilistic combination of broad-spectrum antibiotics. Short-term corticosteroid therapy may be added in the event of threatening cerebral oedema, and anti-epileptic treatment should be systematic in the event of comitiveness, or even prophylactically in the case of any supratentorial location.

Surgical treatment is required in conjunction with medical treatment if the volume of the subdural empyema shows signs of intracranial hypertension or localisation, or if it increases in size under exclusive medical treatment, and its evacuation by trepanation, especially with two holes, is the technique of choice. Craniotomy still has its place, particularly in the event of failure of evacuation by trepanation, but also of 1ère intention in certain teams.
Clinical and CT scan monitoring during treatment is essential, enabling the medical and surgical treatment to be adapted to suit the different situations.
Cerebral entrapment and thrombosis of the dural venous sinuses are the most serious complications of intracranial subdural empyema, and the cause of high mortality.Following early and well-adapted treatment, more than 50% of patients experience a favourable outcome. ?0% of cases of pyogenic subdural empyema in immunocompetent adults. Death generally occurs in complicated forms. The only clearly identifiable prognostic factor with a significant relationship to outcome is the initial state of consciousness. Clinical and CT scan monitoring is essential during follow-up, in order to detect any recurrences, ensure eradication of the infectious site at the site of entry, and ensure compliance with the anti-epileptic treatment systematically instituted in patients who have convulsed, or even prophylactically in the case of supratentorial location of the empyema for certain teams.

In addition :

- We suggest that if there is evidence in favour of a sinus origin of the intracranial subdural empyema (history of sinusitis, presence of purulent rhinorrhoea, presence of a sinus filling, particularly in the frontal sinus on neuroimaging), the probabilistic combination of Cefotaxime and Metronidazole seems sufficient in 1er place.

- We suggest that if there is evidence that the subdural empyema is of otogenic origin (history of chronic otitis media, particularly cholesteatomatous, presence of purulent otorrhea, presence of oto-mastoid filling on neuroimaging), the probabilistic combination of Cefotaxime / Ciprofloxacin / Metronidazole seems more appropriate in 1er place (Pseudomonas possible).

- We suggest that the probabilistic combination of Cefotaxime / Fosfomycin / Metronidazole, which is the most frequent in our series, should only be proposed in 1er cases where there is no data to suggest that the patient should be treated with a combination of Cefotaxime / Fosfomycin / Metronidazole. a particular route of entry, and in cases of post-traumatic origin. Vancomycin can also be used in these cases.

- We suggest that the minimum recommended duration of parenteral antibiotic therapy should be 4 weeks in the case of medico-surgical treatment, and 6 weeks in the case of exclusive medical treatment, and that there are currently no valid recommendations for oral antibiotic therapy.

- We suggest that post-operative scans should always be performed within 24 hours of evacuation of the intracranial subdural empyema.

- We suggest a weekly frequency of scans if medical or surgical treatment is effective, based on the patient's clinical condition and the existence of a significant reduction in the mass effect on the medial structures and in the size of the empyema (:S 2 mm) and regression of the associated cerebral oedema. In other situations, the frequency of check-ups will be decided on a case-by-case basis.

- We suggest that a complete blood count (CBC), together with a blood ionogram and a renal work-up, should be carried out twice weekly in order to detect any haematological, ionic or renal repercussions of antibiotic therapy. Monitoring of the decreasing kinetics of the SV and CRP may be of interest, but seems to contribute little given the existence of many intermediate situations.
- We suggest a monthly schedule of CT scans after patient discharge, with assessment based on the disappearance of subdural empyema or its replacement by CSF and the disappearance of peripheral contrast, with a minimum of one cerebral CT scan without and with injection of contrast medium in the month following discharge.

- Finally, we suggest that anti-epileptic treatment should be systematically continued for at least one year in all patients treated for pyogenic intracranial subdural empyema who have already developed comititude. There is currently no valid recommendation for systematic prophylactic anti-comyema treatment for supratentorial localisations.

BIBLIOGRAPHICAL REFERENCES

1. Passeron H, Sidy Ka A, Diakhate T, Tmbert P. Intracranial suppurations with an otorhinolaryngological portal of entry in children in Senegal. Arch Pediatr. 2010;1?:132-40.

2. Alliez B, Ducolombier A, Gueye L. Collected intracranial suppurations : study of 64 anatomoclinical observations. Med Afr Noire. 1992;39(5):3??-82.

3. Djientcheu VP, Mouafo TF, Esiene A, Kamga YN, Nguefack S, Bello F, et al. Tntracranial suppurations in the African child: a severe but preventable complication. Childs Nerv Syst. 2013;29(1):119-23.

4. Hitchcock E, Andreadis A. Subdural empyema: A review of 29 cases. J Neurol Neurosurg Psychiatry. 1964;2?:422-34.

5. Victor A, Ropper AH. Subdural empyema. J Neurol Neurosurg Psychiatry. 2001;1(1):?49-53.

6. Kubikc S, Adams RD. Subdural empyema. Brain.1943;66:18-42.

?. Djindjian M, Decq P. Abscesses, empyema and spondylodiscitis. Neurochirurgie.1995;3:592-8.

8. Sarrazin JL, Bonneville F, Martin-Blondel G. Cerebral tumours. J Radiol Diagn Tnter. 2012;93(6):503-20.

9. Pal D, Bhattacharyya A, Husain M, Prasad KN, Pandey CM, Gupta RK. Tn vivo proton MR spectroscopy evaluation of pyogenic brain abscesses: a report of 194 cases. Am J Neuroradiol. 2010;31:360-6.

10. Leys D, Petit H. Cerebral abscesses and intracranial empyema. Neurochirurgie. 1994;2:485-91.

11. Debroise A, Bosdure E, Bresson V, Scavarda D, Halbert C, Drancourt M et al. Subdural empyema complicating meningococcal meningitis: a paediatric observation.Arch Pediatr. 2012;19(?):?36-40.

12. Kabré A, Zabsonré SD, Haro Y, Sanou A. Intracranial empyema: clinical, therapeutic and prognostic aspects about 30 cases. Rev CAMES. 2014;2(2):?9-83.

13. Elgamri A, Naja A, Naja T, Elfane M, Hilmani S, Tbahioin K et al. Intracranial empyema. J Neurochirurgie. 2010;6:91-8.

14. Gueye M, Badiane SB, Sakho Y, KoneS, Ba MC, Kabre A. Abscess of the brain and empyema empyema. Dakar Med.1991;36(1):82-?.

15. Loembe M, Okome-Monakou. Intracranial suppurations and empyema in Africa. Med Trop. 199?;5?:186-94.

16. Heckmann JC, Lang CJ, Hartl H, Tomandl B. Multiple brain abscesses caused by Fusobacterium nucleatum treated conservatively. Can J Neurol Sci. 2003;30:266-8.

1?. Hoyt DJ, Fisher SR. Otolaryngologic management of patients with subdural empyema. Laryngoscope. 1991;101:20-4.

18. Yenda K, Mohanty S. Massive falx cerebri empyema Neurol Tndia. 2003;51(1):65-6.

19. Elabbassi SA, Elamraoui F, Chikhaoui N, Kadiri R. Imaging of cerebral suppurations. Maghreb Med. 2000;20(348):22?-30.

20. Tewari MK, Sharma RR, Shuv VK, Lad SD. Spectrum of intracranial subdural empyema in a review of 45 patients. Current surgical options and outcome. Neurol Tndia. 2004;52(3):246-9.

21. Nathoo N, Nadvis S, Van Dellen JR, Gouxs E. Tntracranial subdural empyema in the era of computed tomography: A review of 699 cases. Neurosurgery. 1999;44(3):529-36.

22. Bernardini GL. Diagnosis and management of brain abscess and subdural empyema. Curr Neurol Neurosci Rep. 2004;4(6):448-56.

23. Emery R, Berthelotj B, Ouaheso R. Intracranial abscesses and empyema: neurosurgical management. Ann Fr Anesth Réanim. 1999;18:56?-?3.

24. Kooli T, Loussaief C, Darmoul M, Toumi A, Hattab MN, Chakroun M. Intracranial empyema. Med Mal Tnfect. 2014;44(6):48.

25. Greenlee JE. Subdural empyema. Curr Treat Options Neurol. 2003;5:13-22.

26. Jones NS, Jones T, Walker JL, Bassi S, Punts J. The intracranial complications of rhinosinusitis: can they be prevented? Laryngoscope. 2002;112(1):59-63.

2?. Bannister G, Williams B, Smith S. Treatement of subdural empyema. J Neurosurg. 1981;55:85-8.

28. Hilmani S. Les empyèmes intracrâniens [Thesis]. Medicine: Casablanca; 1995. 185p.

29. Tall A, Beketi A, Loum B, Diallo BK, Wane A, Diop EM et al. Subdural empyema complicating acute frontal sinusitis: 4 cases. Rev Laryngol Otol Rhinol. 2005;2:121-6.

30-Ray S, Riordan A, Tawil M, Mallucci C, Jauhar P, Solomon T et al. Subdural Empyema Caused by Neisseria meningitidis: A Case Report and Review of the Literature.J Pediatr Tnfect Dis. 2016;35(10):1156-9.

31. Dakar A. Les suppurations collectées intracraniennes. J Neurosurgery. 2014;19(3):1?.

32. Furen X, Miong T, Lee T, Ham T, Jui T. Brain abscess: clinical experience and analysis of prognostic factors. Surg Neurol. 2005;6:442-540.

33. Yuen NT, Kuo Y, Ming P, Yen C, Feng C. Community-acquired brain abscess in Taiwan: etiology and probable source of infection. J Microbiol Tmmunol Tnfect. 2004;3?:231-5.

34. Pao-tsuan K, Hiang-kuang T, Chang-pan L, Sheychiang S, Chun-ming L. Brain abscess: clinical analysis of 53 cases. J Microbiol Tnfect. 2003;36:129-36.

35. Calfee DP, Wispelwey B. Brain abscess. Semin Neurol. 2000;20:353-60.

36. Coulibaly HC. Les empyèmes intracrâniens : à propos de 30 observations colligées dans le service de neurochirurgie du CHU Yalgado-Ouedraogo. [Thesis]. Medicine: Ouagadougou; 2012. 120 p.

3?. Zeh OF, Guegang GE, Moifo B, Nguefack S, Nchagnouot MF, Nwatsock JF et al. CT aspects of cerebral complications of bacterial meningitis in children in Yaoundé. Afr J Med Sci. 2014;6(1): 22-9.

38. Zimmerman D, Leeds E, Danziger A. Subdural empyema. Tnd J Radiol Tmaging. 1984;150:41?-22.

39. FuermanT, Wackymp A,Gadeg F,Dubrow T. Craniotomy improves outcome in subdural empyema. Surg Neurol. 1989;32:105-10.

40. Ouiminga HA, Thiam AB, Ndoye N, Fatigba H, Thioub M, Memou S et al. Intracranial empyema: epidemiological, clinical, paraclinical and therapeutic aspects. Retrospective study of 100 observations. Neurosurgery. 2014;60(6):299-303.

41. Bok AP, Peter JC. Subdural empyema: burrholes or craniotomy? A retrospective computerized tomography-era analysis of treatment in 90 cases. Neurosurg. 1993;?8:5?4-8.

42. Delouche A, Attyé A, Grand S, Troprés T, Kastler A, Krainik A. Tntérêt

dela séquence de susceptibilité magnétique en TRM dans l'exploration des traumatismes crâniens légers.Neuroradiol. 2014;41(1):16.

43. Hammami B, Masmoudi M, Charfeddine T, Mnejja M, Ghorbal A. Management of orbital and endocranial complications of acute bacterial sinusitis. J Tun ORL Chir Cerv Faciale. 2014;31:2-6.

44.French H, Schaefer N, Keijzers G, Barison D, Olson S. Tntracranial subdural empyema: a 10-year case series. Ochsner J. 2014;14(2):188-94.

45. Reiner P, Crassard T, Lukaszewicz AC. Cerebral venous thrombosis. Réanimation. 2013;22(6):624-33.

46. Barhmi T, Tazi N, Abada R, Roubal M, Mahtar M. Intracranial complications of frontal sinusitis: about 12 cases. Ann Otolaryngol. 2014;131(4):156.

4?. Scopetta T, Da Rocha AJ, Nunes RH. Meningitis, Empyema, and Brain Abscess in Adults. Am J Roentgenol. 2016;20?(5):141-54.

48. Kaufman DM, Litman N, Miller MH. Sinusitis-induced subdural empyema. Neurology. 1983;33:123-32.

49. Nguefack S, Moifo B, Chiabi A, Mah E, Bogne JB, Fossi M et al. Pasteurella multocida meningitis complicated by brain abscess. Arch Pediatr. 2014;21(3):306-8.

50. Boumediane M. La prise en charge des suppurations Tntracrâniennes : A propos de 1?0 cas au service de Neurochirurgie du CHU Mohamed VT. [Thesis]. Medicine: Marrakech; 2016. 166p.

51. Arlotti M, Grossi P, Pea F, Tomei G. Consensus document on controversial issues for the treatment of infections of the central nervous system: bacterial brain abscesses. Tnt J Tnfect Dis. 2010;14:?9-92.

52. Tsou TP, Lee PT, Lu CY, Chang LY, Huang LM, Chen JM, et al. Microbiology and epidemiology of brain abscess and subdural empyema in a medical center: A 10-year experience. J Microbiol Tmmunol Tnfect. 2009;42:405- 12.

53. Salunke PS, Malik V, Kovai P, Mukherjee KK. Falcotentorial subdural empyema: analysis of 10 cases. Acta Neurochir. 2012;153(1):164-?0.

54. Alimehmeti R, Seferi A, Stroni G, Sallavaci S, Rroji A, Pilika K, et al. Burrhole evacuation for infratentorial subdural empyema. World J Clin Cases. 2013;1:1?2-5.

55. Colpaert C, Van Rompuiy V, Vanderveken O, Venstermans C, Boudewyns A, Menovsky T et al. Tntracranial complications of acute otitis media and Gradenigo's syndrome. B ENT. 2013;9:151-6.

56. Beyneix A. Une médecine du fond des âges: trépanations, amputations et tatouages thérapeutiques au Néolithique. Anthropologie. 2015;119(1) :58-?1.

5?. Tchaleu BC, Luma HN, Mapoure YN, Temfack E, Mankaa EW, Nguemgne C. Exclusive medical treatment of subdural empyema complicating scalp abscess: a case report. Afr Med J. 2015;4(2):55-9.

58. Betz CS, Tssing W, Matschke J, Kremer A, Uhl E, Leunig A. Complications of acute frontal sinusitis: a retrospective study. Eur Arch Otorhinolaryngol. 2008;265(1):63-?2.

59. Mat Nayan SA, Mohd Haspani MS, Abd Latiff AZ, Abdullah JM, Abdullah S. Two surgical methods used in 90 patients with intracranial subdural empyema. J Clin Neurosci. 2009;16(12):156?-?1.

60. Donaldson G, Webster D, Crandon TW. Brain abscess at the University Hospital of the West Tndies. West Tndian Med J. 2000;49:212-5.

62. Hlavinm L, Ratcheson RA. Subdural empyema. Oper Tech Neurosurg. 2000;12:166?-?8.

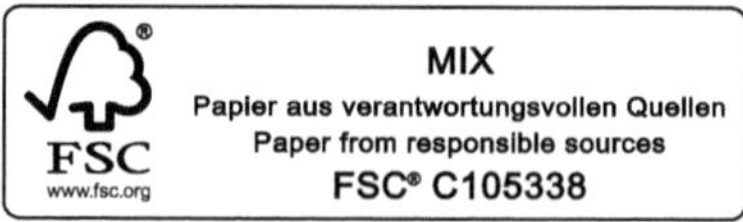

Printed by Books on Demand GmbH, Norderstedt / Germany